AUTOPHAGY

Body's Natural Intelligence for Anti-Aging and Healing - Intermittent Fasting for Weight Loss & Self-Cleansing

FRANCES SPRITZLER

Contents

Introduction

Thank you for purchasing *Autophagy: Body's Natural Intelligence for Anti-Aging and Healing – Intermittent Fasting for Weight Loss & Self-Cleansing*, and congratulations on doing so!

As you begin your journey into understanding this biological and natural process in your body, you will learn some very interesting things about how your body works. When you first learn about what autophagy is, it may sound a little gross, scary, unreal, or strange. Yes, the definition of the name is a little "off," but what it does for your body certainly is not! As you work from chapter to chapter of this book you will find information and advice pulled from various publications and scientific journals. You will learn what the process is, how it works in your body, what the current research reveals, and how you can use it to truly "cleanse" your body.

Using this healthy and natural process, you can help support your general health, boost your immune and metabolic systems, get glowing skin, and lose weight. You can also choose the method for doing this that works for your life! No need to give up all the foods and activities in your life that you enjoy! Instead, small tweaks here and there can make all the difference in how you live your life for years to come. It may sound "simple" or "too good to be true." This is because it is simple to explain, but the mental willpower and determination you need to make these tweaks will make the difference between just reading about how you can take control of your health and weight, and actually embracing it. Once you are done reading this book, hopefully, you are ready to get going!

There are plenty of books on this subject on the market, thanks again for choosing this one! Every effort was made to ensure it is full of as much useful information as possible. Please enjoy!

1

What is Autophagy?

The word "autophagy" is derived from the Ancient Greek word, meaning "hollow" or "self-devouring." It may sound ominous, but it is a natural process in your body to help you regulate the various cellular components you need and do not need for proper functioning. It is descriptive of the process of regulation, and how your body breaks down cells if they are dysfunctional or unnecessary. Those parts that are removed are then recycled or properly disposed of so you can have a healthy body. It is an orderly process or degradation and dissolution.

There are three primary types of autophagy, which occur in your body: chaperone-mediated autophagy, or CMA; microautophagy, and; macroautophagy. Each type has a

1

unique role and purpose in your body. When you are sick or have a disease, your body's response to this stress, which is your body's natural survival instinct, is a response that adapts to the problem at hand. Because of its adaptability, it will either show up and help kill or destroy cells or break them apart to try to restore them. At times, the process can appear to support the morbidity of the affected cells. In cases where your body becomes extremely starved, the natural autophagy process will breakdown parts of cells to help the cell survive on less energy, leading to the best chance of survival. They remove the "unnecessary" components at the moment to help the cells keep up their energy levels.

In 1963, when Dr. Christian de Duve discovered the function of the body's lysosomes, he coined the name, "autophagy." Later, in the 1990s, researchers studying yeast found autophagic-like properties, which lead to the discovery of the process. A Nobel Peace Prize in Physiology or Medicine was awarded in 2016 to Yoshinori Ohsumi, a Japanese researcher who was prominent in the 1990s autophagy deduction. Prior to all of this, in 1962, Keith Porter and a student first observed the process of autophagy at Rockefeller Institute. They identified the lysosome quantity was increased in rat's livers after glucagon was introduced. They observed how some moved to the center of the cells but had a severe flaw in their interpretation—they did not consider the organelles that already existed and the formation of the lysosome. Their name, "autolysis" was coined after Christian de Duve and Alex Novikoff's work, but it was not accurate. This is why de Duve was credited with the discovery in 1963. Christian de Duve began his work after being introduced to a study published in early 1963 by Hruban, Spargo and their colleagues. Their publication described "focal cytoplasm degradation." This observation and study were based off a German study from 1955 studying injuries. Their observations launched de Duve's own inquiry, which ultimately leads to his coining of the process as "autophagy." Not making the same conclusion as Porter and his student, de Duve observed that the function of the lysosome was influenced by the glucagon, but it was a major part of the cellular degradation in the liver of the subjects. During this study, de Duve and his student Russell Deter explained that lysosomes were the reasons for the autophagy caused by glucagon. This is the first moment that lysosomes were described as the center for intracellular autophagy.

After Ohsumi received his award for his work with autophagy, the field grew dynamically throughout the 21st century. Several studies were conducted on the subject, shedding light on new tools for scientists to learn about human's response to disease and their general health. In 1999, Beth Levine and her group of researchers made an incredible discovery that altered the course of autophagy and researchers ever since. Levine and her group identified a strong connection between autophagy and cancer. Even today, the main research topic of autophagy relates to cancer. Another common theme in research is the relationship between immune defense and neurodegeneration. In 2003, the first Gordon Research Conference in Waterville focused on autophagy. Later, in 2005, Daniel Klionsky published a scientific journal focused on autophagy, titled "Autophagy." In 2007, the first Keystone Symposia and Conference held in Monterey was dedicated to autophagy. Research continues to unfold new and interesting applications of understanding about autophagy and its role in the human body.

The Process of Autophagy

All three types of autophagy are facilitated by genes related to autophagy and related enzymes. Because of the size of macroautophagy, it is further divided into "selective" and "bulk" macroautophagy. "Selective" refers to organelle autophagy. This includes ribophagy, coprophagy, pexophagy, lipophagy, and mitophagy. The main type of autophagy in a person's body is Macroautophagy. The primary purpose is to remove damaged organelles from cells or proteins that are not in use. The process works like this: the phagophore selects the items that need to be removed and it surrounds them. This creates an autophagosome, or a double membrane, surrounding the selected organelle or protein. The autophagosome then makes its way through the cell's cytoplasm until it reaches a lysosome. When it finds one, and the two bind together. The autophagosome enters into the lysosome and begins to degrade because of the lysosomal hydrolase.

Other times, the autophagy is more direct, which is known as Microautophagy. The cytoplasm material is engulfed directly into the lysosome. The lysosomal membrane folds inward or is a cellular protrusion called "invagination." A more complex process than the other two is the CMA, or "chaperone-mediated autophagy." The pathway is very specific and involves recognition by a hsc70-containing complex. Basically, this means that when hsc70 complex is present, a protein must have a site that will recognize it. This recognition allows the complex to bind to it, creating CMA-substrate/chaperone complex. This complex then is able to bind to a protein bound for the membrane of the lysosome through the CMA receptor of the protein. This allows the complex to enter the cell. Once inside, the protein unfolds and is sent through the membrane with the help of the hsc70 chaperone. This process is significantly different, mainly because of the translocation of the protein material in a singular manner. It is also an extremely selective process, only allowing very specific material to cross over the barrier of the lysosome.

. . .

Two processes related to Macroautophagy include lipophagy and mitophagy. Lipophagy occurs in both fungus and animals. Autophagy can degrade lipids. In plants, this process is not identifiable yet. Lipid Droplets, or LDs, are the target. These little spheres are the center of most triacyl-glycerols, or TAGs, and are also a single layer of protein for a membrane and phospholipids. This process was observed and defined in 2009 during a study on mice. The other process, mitophagy, is a result of autophagy. When autophagy does its "job," mitochondria can experience selective degradation. This is most commonly observed when the mitochondria are stressed or damaged, making it defective. This process encourages mitochondrial turnover and also stops the dysfunctional mitochondria from piling up. If too much-damaged mitochondria accumulate the cell can begin to degrade. Even if there are healthy mitochondria present alongside dysfunctional mitochondria, the process is still applied to all present in the cell.

The Function of Autophagy

There are several functions of autophagy, including Xeno-phanes, nutrient starvation, infection, programmed cell death, and repair mechanisms. Autophagy is present in a variety of cellular functions for a variety of reasons. Below is a brief synopsis of these functions and how autophagy is involved.

Xenophagy

When an infectious particle enters the body, there is degradation caused by autophagy. This is a term most often applied and found in microbiology. In addition to breaking down an infected particle, this almost-mechanical process of autophagy in your cells is critical to helping your immune system. For example, if your body is attached by an intracellular pathogen such as the bacterium that causes tuberculosis, Mycobacterium tuberculosis, the mechanics and mechanisms that choose what mitochondria to degrade are also responsible for degrading this pathogen.

Nutrient Starvation

Autophagy is present at high levels in yeasts when there is nutrient starvation. This is necessary because the unnecessary proteins are degraded and recycled amino acids are used to synthesize the protein to keep your body alive. An example of this process being present is when an animal severs its ties with its trans-placental food supply after birth. Often in a body that is rich in nutrients form mutant cells of yeast that stop the autophagy process, but when those nutrients deplete, so do these mutant cells. When a body enters into starvation, this process is necessary to help keep the body alive as long as possible. It has been shown in studies with mice and is essential for vacuoles protein degradation when starving.

Infection

Your body has intracellular "danger" receptors, such as Galectin-8, which roam your body looking for trouble. When these receptors sense something is attacking the body, like vesicular stomatitis virus, they begin autophagy on the intracellular pathogens. Galectin-8, for example, binds to the critical vacuole and calls for an autophagy adaptor, like NDP52. This then begins the development of an autophagosome and the degradation of the bacteria.

Programmed Cellular Death

PCD, or "programmed cellular death," is related to the look of the autophagosome and relies on the protein in autophagy. This often is associated with a specific process, which is now called "autophagic PCD." There is still debate, much like the "chicken and the egg," about whether cell death caused this process or if this process caused the death of the cell. The process could be an attempt to repair the cell, or an attempt to stop cellular death, or it could be the reason the cell is dying. To this day, there are no histochemical or morphological studies that show the cause in the relationship between the death of the cell and the activity of autophagy in it. What was previously the favored opinion, that autophagy was actually causing the cells to die, has fallen in popularity as more evidence leans towards the possibility of the process trying to save the cell. For example, some arguments present insect metamorphosis as an example of a form of PCD that shows how the cells can be saved instead of killed. It is a distinct cellular change that no other example has shown. After a viral infection, the degree, and type of stress that signals for regulation can determine the chances of a cell of survival or death. These recent studies still need more research to show this relationship; however, the biochemical and pharmacological results are promising.

Repair Mechanism

The reason you age is that your body stops removing damaged cells, but rather allows them to accumulate in your body. This is why you begin to get wrinkles and your muscles begin to breakdown. Degeneration of autophagy is credited as one of the reasons for this cellular accumulation. This is because a working autophagic process breaks down the dysfunctional proteins, cell membranes, and organelles. If your body decides to no longer use this process, you begin to start aging. When there are lysosomal damage autophagy receptors, like by "directors" Galectin-8 and Galectin-3, and autophagy is present. When this is triggered, galectins often call for help from other receptors like NDP52 and TRIM16. This also directly impacts AMPK and mTOR activity in your body. AMPK and mTOR, on the other hand, activate and also inhibit autophagy respectively in your body.

2

How Autophagy Works

A Phagaphore is the "hallmark" of the autophagy process. It is a double-membrane structure that moves around. Unlike secretory transport vesicles that separate from an organelle carrying "cargo" inside already, the phagophore picks up its load while it is assembling. The sequential expansion allows the phagophore to take on a little load or a large load. There is a lot of flexibility in how much they can carry. When it expands to load in something, it separates the cytoplasmic parts, including other, complete organelles, lipids, and proteins. As soon as it is loaded, it closes and turns into an autophagosome. Once matured into the autophagosome, the cargo remains contained in the lumen. Through-membrane fusion the autophagosome delivers its load to the lytic compartments. In plants and fungi, this is vacuole and in metazoans it is lysosomes. Once there, the cargo is degraded and recycled.

It is possible to see autophagy broadly categorized into two categories—nonselective and selective. It is categorized by what is being picked up or "eaten." When studied more extensively, it is broken down further into macroautophagy, microautophagy, and CMA, or chaperone-mediated Autophagy, as described in the previous chapter. In order for the cells in your body to be in balance or in homeostasis, autophagy must be present and functioning properly. In addition, autophagy is necessary for cellular survival when your body is stressed, such as when it is nutrient deficient. The process of autophagy is upregulated. This means that the degradation and sequestering of parts of the cell are determined by the severity of the situation. Once it arrives and assesses the "damage," the process returns macro-molecules into the cytosol. This is essential to the metabolic reaction of the cell and generates power and energy.

The process of autophagy is precisely orchestrated and tightly regulated. The pathological and physiological role it plays in your body is essential, as evidenced by its support in the health of your cells both when your body is under stress, like starvation or infection, and while healthy. It has been found that this process is also critical during the development of mammals. It is a vital modulator of a number of disorders and diseases as well. The role of the pathway is better understood when you understand autophagy's involvement in both human development and diseases. The implication of this knowledge can be used to more effectively treat disease as well as support general health. While it is now understood how the process works from a general function and morphology, the pathway is intricate and the exact steps in the process are still being discovered.

Autophagy Mechanisms

Large molecules are broken down in cells through multiple catabolic pathways. One of the most notable pathways is the collaboration of ubiquitin, a small protein, with an additional cellular protein. After, this typically leads to more ubiquitin molecules to create a chain of polyubiquitin. This releases amino acids, using proteasome to mark the protein for degradation. Other, similar mechanisms for degradation exist with additional biological polymers. For example, this process exists for lipids and carbohydrates as well.

There are two reasons why autophagy is unique: first, it is able to select what and how much cargo it wants to carry, and, second, it is very flexible. It can encourage degradation for a substantial variety and number of substrates, allowing cells to rapidly and effectively recycle the materials used in basic cellular building. This is especially important in the face of nutrient deficiency. In addition, the pathway of autophagy is the single one able to degrade an entire organelle. It can do this in a targeted manner or at random. The complicated setting for eukaryotic cells is balanced by this crucial process.

The process is very regulated, only releasing and increased when necessary. It is also tightly monitored so it can respond in a timely fashion. The TOR complex 1, or a cell's main metabolic sensor, is highly aware of how much amino acids and growth factors are present. It prevents autophagy when there is an abundance of these in the cell. When there are not enough of these present in the cell, the TOR complex 1 is turned "off," and autophagy is allowed to increase. While this is happening, additional molecular regulators keep an eye on cells for the levels of various nutrients, like glucose, or ATP energy. When the receptors sense that these items are low, they trigger autophagy.

Once autophagy begins, multiple proteins related to autophagy, called Atg, come together to create the phagophore and the next steps of autophagy. In the 1990s, the ATG genes of yeast were discovered. This discovery altered the course of autophagy research and the understanding of the process forever. Prior to this discovery, autophagy was just a generic description of the process.

After this, science understood that the process is a major mechanism occurring at the molecular level. Autophagy's primary mechanism was further defined in a study using Saccharomyces cerevisiae, budding yeast that is genetically tractable. After this, more research in other organisms has followed. This spiral of discovery showed the world the conservative evolution in the function and nature of the machinery in autophagy in all living forms—from humans to yeast.

Scientists are fairly clear about the process of autophagy, but the puzzle is far from being completed. There are still many missing pieces to the overall picture of autophagy. For example, it still remains to be established by autophagosome's membrane donor. In addition, scientists still cannot determine precisely how regulations of the expansion of the phagophore are accomplished. It is not understood how frequent autophagosome is generated. Additional questions come up when scientists look at the various types of autophagy and its selectivity as well as the mystery of the triggering and regulation process. Human disease, healthy development and growth, and development of embryos have all been linked to the autophagy process; hence, uncovering more information about the process is vital for human homeostasis.

. . .

When Autophagy Goes Wrong

Cancer, neurodegenerative disorders, and infectious disease are pathologies all linked to the deregulation of the autophagy process. As more research is produced, it is becoming more evident that the relationship between disease and autophagy is vital to creating more effective therapies and interventions for some of the worst human diseases impacting our society today.

Yasuko Rikihisa of the College of Veterinary Medicine at Virginia Tech, first reported the induction of autophagy in 1984. The study produced showed that when incubated mammalian cells were infected with a tick-borne illness, rickettsiae, the cells triggered autophagosomes to be formed. Unfortunately, the understanding of this process on eukaryotic cells has just begun. Part of this process has shown to limit inflammation. Inflammation is critical to helping the body heal from infection or disease, but extended inflammation can cause tissue damage and other diseases. These preliminary findings suggest that in addition to monitoring the elimination of pathogens, it can also prevent unnecessary tissue degradation by limiting the presence of inflammation at the site.

At the Weill Cornell Medical College, J. Magarian Blander discovered that autophagy is vital to the stress response pathway of a cell when there is an infection present. The autophagy process is necessary for triggering the immune response after the stress is found in an infected cell. But at the Jan Lunemann's lab at the University of Zurich, it was discovered that it was not always helpful to modulate the immune system through autophagy. The process of autophagy may actually aggravate diseases like multiple sclerosis, or MS, which is an autoimmune disease impacting the central nervous system. Nerve degeneration and autoimmune disease is still an uncertain area for autophagy.

It is clear, however, that one of the main roles of autophagy is protection against several neurodegenerative disorders, like Parkinson's Disease and Huntington's Disease. One of the main culprits that lead to Huntington's disease—the mutant HTT, an aggregation-prone protein—is degraded through autophagy, according to the research published by David Rubinsztein and his colleagues at the Cambridge Institute for Medical Research. With regard to Parkinson's disease, reduction of mitophagy is a primary reason for pathogenesis. This is not surprising and the understanding that homeostasis of mitophagy is necessary for healthy neurological functioning.

Cancer is also connected to autophagy. The Levine Group discovered in 1999 that mice with only one autophagy-related gene, Becn-1, had more tumors. Research has shown that autophagy is critical in preventing tumor creation and also in stopping malignancy in present tumors. The generation and progression of tumors have several factors that respond to this dual role autophagy plays in the process. Tumors are prevented because autophagy suppresses the known stressors that cause tumor growth, such as mitochondrial dysfunction, metabolic disruption, and genomic instability. But once a tumor is created, the "playing field" changes dramatically. Growth and proliferation of a cell with a tumor have more metabolic demands than a healthy cell. But because of cancer, the vasculature cannot supply it with the necessary nutrients. This means the cell relies on upregulating autophagy to meet its growing needs. This means that inhibiting autophagy can actually help "starve" cancer cells. The challenge scientists face with this knowledge is the balance necessary for tumor starvation without also causing neurodegeneration and increasing the likelihood of infection. Because the process is not straightforward and autophagy is still being revealed, it is important the therapies using autophagy for cancer treatment are approached with extreme care.

The study of autophagy is still underway and a popular field for exploration. It is exciting is for science to explore because of the many benefits it provides to our bodies. It plays a critical role in our health and wellbeing. While some crucial and beneficial mechanics have been revealed over the last several decades, understanding of autophagy is still in its early stages. Things related to the initiation, progression, and regulation have provided the present understanding of autophagy, but there are still many questions that scientists are looking to answer. In fact, many would say there are still more questions than answers, especially regarding proteins related to autophagy. Therapeutic intervention, in particular, is looking into the role autophagy plays in the process of pathophysiology. It is interesting to recognize that a person's instinctual need to eat to stay alive extends beyond the need to consume food, but it includes the need to eat oneself, at least, on a cellular level.

3

The Benefits of Autophagy

I t may sound a bit ominous to say that you are eating yourself, but the reality is that your cells are doing this all the time inside of you. And the purpose is to help repair or remove damaged cells so you can live a healthy and balanced life. Some even claim that this process is the secret to a long life, even the "fountain of youth," if you will. When you need to save energy, fight away an infection, or heal damage, your body begins the autophagy process. This chapter outlines 12 of the most common and beneficial reasons you want autophagy in your life and working right.

1. It can help save your life.

This may sound a little dramatic, but it is true. This biological response has one primary purpose—to save you.

Anytime something compromises your life at a cellular level, autophagy is triggered to stop it. This includes when your body is extremely stressed, you are invaded by infection, or when you are starving. The process seeks to minimize any damage and repair as much as possible. You can use this known and natural process in collaboration with other ancient healing techniques, like intermittent fasting where your body relies on fat for fuel and not glucose. This combination activates autophagy to help stave off infections, lower inflammation, and heal the damage caused by inflammation and infection. Glucose is an intruder and known invader. Inflammation is known to inhibit your immune system from functioning properly in the locations being inflamed. Because of autophagy, humans and almost all living beings have and still can use autophagy to conserve their energy and repair problems, especially in times where energy is not readily available. It is also a vital piece of the body's immune system and your ability to fight disease and reduce the risk of developing cancer.

2. It can help you live a longer and more full life.

While the research is still being conducted in the area of this benefit, preliminary findings show that there are anti-aging benefits to autophagy as well. It may sound "too good to be true," but the benefits do not just stop at skin-level. Your cellular health is improved with a fast-acting and efficient autophagy response in your body. Cells do not simply bring in nutrients all the time; sometimes they degrade and remove parts that no longer work for them. They self-heal by recycling damage or removing toxins from their entity. As your body heals itself, the cells begin to function more efficiently. While they may be older cells, they have new energy and begin acting more like a newer cell. This can be used to explain why some people look much younger than their chronological age. Their biology suggests that they are much younger. The fewer toxins your body has to fight back, and how efficient your body is at healing itself, the younger your cells, and your overall body look.

3. It helps your metabolism function more efficiently.

Your cells generate energy from mitochondria. They are the components that burn fat and create ATP or your body's currency for energy. Autophagy removes or helps replace parts of a cell, such as the mitochondria. As the mitochondria create energy, it leaves behind a lot of toxic build up. This can lead to cellular damage. Autophagy is a proactive process to help break the residue early to prevent the preventable "wear and tear" on your cells. In addition, the process of autophagy on other parts of the cell encourages the rest of the cell to work properly as well. It means that when it works more efficiently your cells create protein as well as burn off fuel. The healthier your cells are, the better you are at burning fuel sources. This means you have a more efficient and effective body.

4. It lowers your risk of developing a neurodegenerative disease.

The proteins that are in your brain and around it begin to stop working correctly. They are not folded correctly and end up resulting in disease in your brain. This is a long time process, but the malfunction begins at a much earlier age. When your body is functioning properly, autophagy removes the proteins that are not working right. This means that these defective proteins do not have the ability to accumulate and build up, leading to these diseases. For example, Parkinson's disease requires autophagy to remove the a-synuclein and Alzheimer's disease requires it to remove amyloid. Both are malfunctioning proteins. When you have constantly high blood sugar, your body cannot remove the "clutter" that builds up around your brain. This is why many medical professionals recognize the connection between diabetes and dementia. Autophagy cannot activate when you have a lot of glucose, allowing this build up to occur. Stabilize blood sugar and you can clear more dysfunction, supporting your brain health.

5. It can help stabilize inflammation.

. . .

Not all inflammation is bad. Your body needs to send fluid and swelling to places that are damaged or infected to help isolate the damage before it can be cleared up. The problem lies when inflammation becomes a chronic condition. This starts to wreak havoc on your tissues and body. It leads to a host of illnesses and diseases. When your body is functioning properly, and autophagy can do its job, it creates the "just right" situation of inflammation in your body. It supports the triggering response for inflammation—either encouraging the inflammation or squashing it. For example, when there are invaders and inflammation is necessary, autophagy helps pass along the message that inflammation is necessary. In fact, it is autophagy that alerts your immune system that it needs to attack and just how it needs to do it. On the other hand, autophagy is also responsible for telling your immune system to lower your inflammation. Antigens are the proteins that are released to your immune system to trigger inflammation. When your cells do not need the inflammation, autophagy removes those signals.

6. It helps fight off infectious diseases.

As mentioned previously, your immune system is recruited when autophagy calls for it. Viruses or microbes that reside in cells, such as HIV or Mycobacterium, can also be directly removed through autophagy. This is because it is a flexible and adaptive process that can take on small and large loads to support the health of your cells. In addition, when you suffer from an infection, it leaves behind various levels and kinds of toxins in your body. Autophagy removes these toxins. This is particularly helpful to you with food-borne illnesses.

7. It helps your muscles perform better.

Muscles need to be repaired after you work them out. The process of "building" muscle is actually an attack on the muscle, inflaming it and creating little micro-tears. This inflammation and tearing need to be healed. In addition, during exercise, you need more energy. Your body responds at a cellular level by triggering autophagy. It first begins by lowering the amount of energy necessary to work that targeted muscle. It then removes the damaged parts and helps bring homeostasis to your energy with the intention of preventing further damage to the area.

8. It helps prevent cancerous cells from forming.

The best way to treat a disease is to prevent the disease. This is especially true for cancer. Pro-cancer responses in your body, such as the response to damaged DNA, unstable genomes, and chronic inflammation, are suppressed with autophagy. In a study on mice that were genetically engineered to have a lower-functioning autophagy process, they experienced a significantly higher rate of cancer development than those with an average autophagy process. Once cancer develops, it can use the autophagy process to gather more fuel for its rapid growth and also "hide" from your immune system. More research on this relationship between cancer and autophagy is being conducted and necessary to make significant breakthroughs in more effective therapeutic options for those at risk and suffering from cancer. Additionally, it is still hazy how much damage chemotherapy-affected non-cancerous cells have on the process and activation of autophagy. More research is being conducted and necessary to identify if the damage of chemotherapy on cancer cells— by killing them directly—is better for you and your overall health than the ability of your own cells to handle the invasion. For example, if you could trigger autophagy to attack and treat those affected cells, is that a better treatment option than introducing chemotherapy? The results of this research could be revolutionary for cancer treatment in the future.

9. It can help your digestion and digestive health.

Your gastrointestinal tract's cells in the lining are always working. Actually, if you are very curious, you can examine your feces and see that the majority of your excrement is actually made up of your own cells! When your GI tract triggers autophagy, those cells are restored, repaired, and cleared out of toxins that they do not need. They also alert your immune system to turn on or off as needed. Chronic inflammation in your bowel is a common illness to battle. This is typically in response to a chronic trigger for your immune system to work in your GI tract. Having this constantly working ends up overwhelming your bowels, which means you need to be able to support this always-working system by giving it a chance to rest, repair, and renew. For example, giving your bowel an extended break from digesting food so it can properly trigger autophagy and heal itself is a great benefit you can encourage during intermittent fasting or fasting periods.

10. It can help clear and support the health of your skin.

Your skin is the largest organ in your body and it is the one that also interfaces with the world around you. This means it is directly and immediately impacted by things like physical damage when something touches it, changes to the humidity levels, cold or hot temperatures, light, air pollution, and chemicals. Skin takes on a lot of damage and needs constant repair from the top of your head to the bottoms of your feet. When skin cells have accumulated toxins or damage, they stay where they are and they age. Your skin cells are constantly being replaced without autophagy, but the process of autophagy is necessary for helping heal and repair your existing ones. This helps the skin stay young and "glow." Because of the skin cell's interaction with exterior influence, there is a greater opportunity for them to collect bacteria that can lead to serious damage to your body. The best way to support your skin cells is to take care of your skin from the inside and out. The more you support your autophagy process, the better your skin will look and feel.

11. It helps you maintain or achieve a healthy weight.

There are several reasons your autophagy process supports a healthy weight. Here is a quick list of a few of those reasons;

- Autophagy protects your protein but burns your fat for fuel. If you are fasting for an extended period of time, you will lose mass from protein loss, but shorter fasts trigger autophagy to burn your fat stores for energy and protect your protein levels. This means you will settle into healthier weight for your body type.
- Autophagy stops unnecessary and chronic inflammation. Chronic inflammation triggers your body to store energy because of the increase in insulin. As you lower your insulin levels through autophagy, the less inflammation you have, allowing your weight to find a healthy balance.
- Autophagy lowers the toxin levels present in your cells. If you can get the toxins out of your body, the fewer fat cells you need to store the "baggage."

- Autophagy helps your metabolism be more efficient. It encourages this efficiency by healing cellular parts that create and "package" proteins and create energy. This is very helpful when your cells switch from burning glucose for energy instead of fat.

12. It minimizes the deaths of your cells.

There is a term often confused with autophagy, apoptosis. Autophagy is about self-consumption of cells, while apoptosis is cellular death. Unlike autophagy, cellular death is messy and leaves behind garbage that needs to be cleaned up. Your body triggers inflammation to go to the site and get it back to working order. If you can prevent your cells from dying this messy death by encouraging repair or clean removal, the less effort your body requires to clean up and create new cells. In addition, you will minimize unnecessary inflammation by self-eating instead of destroying. Reducing the number of cellular deaths allows that energy to be reallocated to help create new cells that have a higher turnover, like your GI tract or your skin. Not all cells require constant replacement, so the more you can repair the existing ones, the more you allow your body to spend its energy elsewhere, the better your health will be.

4

How to Activate Autophagy

Y ou may be onboard with the idea of having your cells
eat each other, but are probably now wondering how
you would go about doing it. Or more accurately, how you
would trigger your body to kick start this process for you.
The good news is that autophagy is a response to stress. This
means that when you stress your body in certain ways, the
process is triggered. But not all stress will do the trick. When
you add a little bit extra stress to your body, the self-
consumption process is elevated. This added stress can be
uncomfortable at the moment, but the idea is that this little
bit of extra stress can lead to incredible, long-term joy.
Adding more stress in a controlled manner can result in
amazing benefits to your body. There are three primary
ways to induce your autophagy process; exercise, fasting,
and decrease your carbohydrate intake significantly.

Exercise

You have probably heard for a long time now that diet and exercise are the keys to a long and healthy life. This is no different, and the science to back up this is here for you in the first and second chapters. Exercise stresses your body at the moment. This is why people have pains after a hard workout, grunt when it is challenging, and sweat. Working out your muscles is actually damaging them, as introduced in the previous chapter. When your muscles work hard, they get little tears in them that need to be repaired. Your body responds to these tears quickly, and while repairing the damage you just did, the body makes the muscle stronger so it can resist any future "damage" you might inflict upon it. You may not think of exercising as a way to clean out your cellular build up or toxins, but its one of the most common and popular ways to renew your cells. This helps explain why you feel so fresh and rejuvenated after a good, hard workout.

In one study on mice with highlighted autophagosomes, the researchers found that after they ran on a treadmill for 30 minutes their autophagy process was dramatically increased. An autophagosome is a resulting structure in the autophagy process. It forms around the damaged or toxic part of the cell and removes it to be disposed of, leaving behind the healthy parts of the cell. The increase in exercise provided evidence that these became more efficient and frequent than when the mice for less active. And it did not just increase the rate of autophagy while exercising! The increased rate of self-consumption continued for 80 minutes after stopping exercise. While there are no concrete studies or information regarding how much or how often a human should exercise to increase autophagy, it is clear the relationship exists in humans as well. Dr. Daniel Klionsky, a University of Michigan cellular biologist, explains that it is hard to deter-mine the level of exercise a human must undergo to trigger their autophagy process, but there are so many clear benefits to exercise that no matter what you do, it will help support your body on some level. The best assumption to make in this case is to engage in more intense exercise regimens a few times a week for the best results. This is for general health benefits, but will also be the best amount of controlled stress on your body to trigger your autophagy.

Fasting

Cleanses that introduce any form of food or drink besides water into the body will actually prevent the trigger of autophagy, not allowing the body to effectively cleanse itself of toxins, as desired on a cleanse. Instead, simply skipping a meal or two or three can be the best stress on the body that triggers autophagy, offering a true cleanse. Your body will probably not like it at the moment, but the benefits will be something it will enjoy for a long time. Research has shown, over and over again, that engaging in an occasional fast can help you lower risks of various illnesses like heart disease and diabetes. The reason for these benefits that medical professionals and scientists claim is because of autophagy.

There are several studies that have been published that specifically look at fasting, autophagy, and brain health. It is clear there is a distinct connection between lowering the risk of developing a neurodegenerative disease, like Parkinson's disease or Alzheimer's disease, when you engage in short-term fasts. Other studies reveal that intermittent fasts help support proper brain function, brain structure, and neuro-plasticity. This is what helps your brain learn new information easier. While this information is exciting, it is not completely clear if autophagy is the reason and most of these studies are conducted on animals. While the benefits are promising, they are not always applicable to human subjects.

There are a variety of adaptations for intermittent fasting, and it is something that can fit into almost anyone's life because of this. You can choose to abstain from eating food anywhere between 12 to 36 hours in a stretch, always drinking a lot of water during the fast. You can also engage in moderate to light physical activity during this time to help your body upregulate the results, but it is not typically advisable to engage in intense workouts during a fasting period. In addition, you can choose to fast only during certain times of the year, a certain day of the month, or one or more days a week.

Decrease Your Intake of Carbohydrates

Fasting on a regular basis can be a challenge for many people, especially if you are used to constantly eating. In addition, this is contradictory to a lot of popular advice available now, encouraging people to eat little meals consistently throughout the day to boost metabolism. What research has shown, however, is that eating constantly does not keep your metabolism and hunger "satisfied," but rather creates a constant "hunger" hormone that keeps you wanting to eat and eat. Instead, when you fast, you learn the difference between true hunger and a triggered response at the time you normally eat a meal. You break your body of these habits and encourage it to focus on your cellular repair and fat-fuel burning instead. If you are having trouble getting into an intermittent fasting schedule, you can mimic the benefits in another way by decreasing your intake of carbohydrates.

This similar process is called ketosis. A lot of people who work out regularly or are looking to improve their long-term health and well-being have been turning to this type of eating regimen. The concept aims to significantly reduce the carbs that are consumed so your body must use the fat for fuel instead of injected glucose from the conversion of the carbs. When your body enters into ketosis, it mirrors a lot of the same changes to your metabolism that autophagy offers. You get to enjoy the benefits of fasting without having to complete fast. In addition to the similar benefits to your metabolism, ketosis has been shown to help you maintain healthy body weight, protect your muscle mass, prevent and fight tumors, lower your risk of type-2 diabetes, minimize the risk of neurological diseases, and treat some brain disorders, like epilepsy. For example, in one recent study, more than 50% of the children with epilepsy that followed this diet experienced more than half the frequency of seizures than their peers not following the diet.

In addition to removing a lot of the carbs, you increase your intake of healthy fat. Most of your calories, up to 70%, come from fat on the Keto diet. This means eating a lot of meat, avocado, peanut butter, to name a few. Protein is up to 30% of your daily caloric intake. If you have room for carbs, you need to keep them to less than 50 grams every day. This is an extreme diet that many people ease into over time. If you can, being with a mix of fat/protein/carbs with your carb intake not exceeding 30% of your daily caloric intake and work back from there. Some find this regimen of eating more challenging than fasting, so it is wise to look into and try out what method works best for you in triggering your autophagy response.

If you are still looking at these three primary methods for triggering autophagy and wondering if there are other, easier ways, you will be discouraged to find that there are none. There will be a lot of money when researchers find a way to trigger autophagy or mimic it in a synthetic form like a pill, and it is being researched and considered now, but this is a long way off. Until the process is better understood, it is not possible to chemically induce the process in a human body. It is also unwise to turn to synthetic and chemical methods to avoid dieting and exercise for your wellbeing. It is also important to note that there are anti-epilepsy drugs being developed to mirror the state of ketosis in the body. If those become available, it is probable that people will begin taking them to mimic autophagy in the body instead of approaching it through traditional diet and exercise methods.

Keep in mind that the process of ketosis in the body is complex, as the process of autophagy. The idea that a single pill can mimic this entire, intricate and complex process is unrealistic. The stress required to enter ketosis, for example, may be an integral part of the process. This means you will need to still exert effort and energy to get the pill to work, in any form. It is also likely that the pill will only encourage one or two of the benefits of ketosis for a person suffering from epilepsy, and not target any other benefits of ketosis. Yes, the three methods of activating autophagy and ketosis listed above all require effort and it is important to also remember that you do not need to do each of them every day to get the results and benefits. Just a couple of hours a week or month can do the trick for supporting your cellular health.

Finally, there are plenty of published research available to show the indication of the various benefits of autophagy as well as how to activate it in a healthy way. The little bit of short-term and controlled stress can lead to controlled and systematic self-destruction so you can end up living a longer, healthier life. It is an ancient survival process that is designed to help the body in times of stress, like when your ancestors had to go days between meals that they hunted to feed themselves and their family. Starvation and physical exertion have the ability to kill you, but over millions of years, human bodies have evolved to turn those "bad" situations into something that can actually help you.

5

Extended Water Fasting

If you want to greatly improve your health and life, you can turn to this ancient strategy for healing and health; water fasting. Keep in mind; however, this process requires practice, patience, and strategy. You do not want to begin this fasting method without prior planning and research. You need to understand what the results can be, what it does to your body, and what can happen if you are not carefully monitoring your progress.

The first thing you need to know is why you should consider fasting. There are many different benefits to fasting. For starters, it is the absolute best method for controlling your insulin and glucose levels. Even better than medicine! One of the best measures for a healthy, long, and meaningful life is your glucose levels. If you can keep these controlled, you can expect to live a healthy, long life. You want your body to run on its own energy source, fat cells, not on spikes of insulin and glucose. If you keep these levels low and stable, your body will keep using its own fuel for energy. Also, fasting helps to keep testosterone levels even. When you eat, your testosterone levels lower, which is what triggers an increase in insulin and glucose. This, in turn, increases inflammation and ultimately aging of your cells. When you establish a lasting habit, your body changes its relationship with food. You recognize that you do not "need" food all the time to stay active and healthy. Your body discovers, or rather re-discover, that it is able to maintain a healthy level of glucose and fuel itself with its fat stores.

Another benefit of fasting is autophagy itself. When autophagy increases, so do a host of health benefits in your body, as described in the previous chapter. This response to fasting can lead to amazing and "miraculous" changes to your body, like improved skin appearance and texture, shrinking cancer, and cured diseases, among others. One researcher found that engaging in a water-only fast for four days can help reset your immune system. Some people need a longer fast, especially in the beginning, while others can do it for only a day or two to experience the benefits. It is best to work with a medical professional and closely observe your body during this time to make sure it is reaching its optimal reset. As you age, your blood begins to accumulate a lot of T-cells. Each one is programmed to fight a certain microbe. But the problem is that these T-cells have been programmed, and you do not have enough "student" T-cells that can learn to adapt to new problems. This compromises your immune system. When you fast, however, you give your body time to remove the unnecessary cells and rebuild your immune system with the "student" T-cells.

The third benefit of extended water fasting is epigenetics. This means the process of changing the "bad" genes into "good" ones, encouraging the "good" genes to do more, and turning off "bad" ones that cannot or will not convert. Anytime you fast, your genes start to shift back to their natural, beginning state. They are changed into healthier versions of themselves and also positively impact your dietary choices. This can occur during a single day fast or during extended fasts, but the more frequent you fast and support the natural and healthy state of your genes, the better benefits you can experience.

The final benefit of extended water fasting includes hormone sensitivity. You can really experience the shift in your hormones when you fast. One particular hormone that you can notice a change in is your growth hormone. During a fasting period, you are not creating more hormones, but rather, becoming more sensitive and aware of the ones you have. Any hormone connected to your health and healing is dramatically increased during fasting periods.

In addition to being clear about what you can experience when you fast, it is clear about why you want to fast. It is important to be clear about why you want to trigger autophagy. For some people, it is to lose weight but for others, it is to support their health. Take a moment to be honest about your intentions with autophagy and fasting, so that as you begin your process, you know how to monitor your progress and success accurately. For example, if your goal is to support your general health and minimize the risk for cancer and other diseases, tracking your weight is not the best gauge for success. If you are looking to find and maintain a healthy weight, monitoring your hormones may not be the best use of your time. Your "why" can be deeper as well. Many people turn to autophagy and fasting to prolong their life so they can be a meaningful part of their family for a longer period of time. Others do it to control a disease that they have been diagnosed with. And still, others fast for religious reasons.

The task of extended water fasting is a challenge. It is best to begin the preparation for this type of autophagy trigger by mentally preparing for the timeframe. There will be a time when it feels like your body and your mind are aligning to beg you for food. It is stressed and operating in uncharted territory. You are breaking long-held habits and patterns, which is stressful. But remember, when you hit day three and you are longing for a big meal, that this stress and it leads to amazing benefits later. You need to mentally prepare ahead of time for this temptation and challenge. How will you plan on overcoming these urges in a healthy manner? This temptation and desire will occur for a day or two and then you can expect to have a shift in perception. Your mindset changes and your mental acuity are returned.

You are no longer obsessed with food but are rather turned away by the idea of it. At this point, your body has realized that it is operating better now without the glucose-fueled energy it was used to before. Prepare yourself to get through the "tough times" so you can get to this state.

While you are on your extended water fast, it is advisable to prepare for changes to your mental alertness. Before starting, you may have some "brain fog." You could experience trouble concentrating and remembering things. When you are fasting, your alertness may be enhanced. You feel more focused and engaged. You have a better memory. It is like the fog is lifted. Prepare to experience a dip in this process. However, as you enter into the phase where your body and mind are asking for food, your mental acuity could be limited. You may find yourself constantly distracted, having trouble focusing on anything other than food, and being forgetful. This is your body adjusting. Once you leave this phase, you will return to this clear and focused mental awareness that you experienced before. It can seem like a dramatic swing each time, but when you experience the clarity, you will know what stage you are dealing with.

It is also important to consider the weight loss you will experience rapidly. When you fast you can expect to drop large amounts of weight quickly. You are also experiencing a removal of toxins that have been stored for a long time in your body, particularly deep in your tissues. The good news is that your body will not drop into unhealthy territory right away. In fact, it will drop down rapidly to a healthy weight balance and sit there. If you find you drop weight and then it stagnates for a while at a certain number, chances are that weight is where you need to be for your body's homeostasis. As you continue to fast, you will see fluctuations in your weight still, but not as dramatic once you reach your balance. This is in part because your body instinctively knows that it needs to remove the affected tissue and dysfunctional DNA but leave the healthy muscle alone. When you do this, medical professionals are in awe about how your body will eat a tumor while fasting. Endometriosis, a reproductive issue involving scar tissue, is also consumed while fasting and as autophagy is increased. Other benefits you can experience include cleared congestion and better breathing patterns.

It is also possible for others to experience weight gain. As you heal your gut, your body can then begin to build muscle like it was not able to do previously. As you increase hormones like your growth hormone, estrogen, and testosterone, you can expect your body to absorb food better. This can lead to weight gain for those that need it in order to reach a more balanced, healthy weight. Bodybuilders use this fasting then feasting method to help them rapidly gain weight in muscle mass.

You can track your levels during a fast to make sure things are progressing as they should. For example, you should be able to see that your glucose levels are dropping down low and that ketones are rising. Ketones are necessary for you to enter into ketosis, a benefit described in the previous chapter. Glucose needs to be minimal in your body so that your cells switch to using fat as a fuel source instead. You can track your levels with blood, urine, or saliva testing kits. Ketones should remain anywhere from 0.5 mmol/L and 5.0 mmol/L so your body is functioning properly in ketosis. Some people can operate at a healthy level with ketones as high as 7.0 mmol/L; however, you do not want them to rise about 8.0 mmol/L. For glucose, you want your numbers in the 60s if your ketones are above 3.0 mmol/L. This "sweet spot" is what most people believe and see as the best place for bad cell removal and repair. If you can get to this balance between ketones and glucose you can be sure that your body is functioning optimally.

During your extended water fast, make time for rest. You may experience a dip in energy, especially in the beginning days, but you will probably still feel a good amount of energy. Be careful not to overexert yourself during this time, though. Exercise on extended water fast will do more harm than good right now. Your stores of protein are healing and exercise can damage this process. Minor to moderate activity is ok, but try to avoid anything too aggressive. Give your body the time it needs to restore itself by taking it easy during this time.

The concept is simple, do not eat anything, and drink plain water only. Maybe sprinkle a little sea salt for something different, but try not to introduce in anything that can kick in your metabolism. But while it is simple to grasp, applying it and sticking to it is not. Like preparing for the "hard days," when your body and mind are asking for a big, greasy meal, you need to remember that most of this is a mental game. You have habits and neuropathways that have been ingrained for a long time that you are altering. It is not wrong, but it does take control. Bringing in a support team to help keep you motivated can do wonders when your mind is struggling. Maybe this is a significant other who is cheering on you, or a "partner in crime," who is doing it along with you. It can be your healthcare professional or any person who will help you stay on the course. You need to make the commitment, stick to it, rely on your support system, and be clear about your purpose. And if you fail, just give it another try. Every little step you make towards supporting your health is beneficial, so just keep going!

6

Intermittent Fasting

There are several studies on the benefits and effects of intermittent fasting on the body. There are several different "kinds" of intermittent fasting, but one of the most common is fasting from 12 to 36 hours one or more days during the week. The process of autophagy is vital to the homeostasis of living organisms at a cellular level, and it has been found in various living entities including humans, bugs, animals, fungi, plants, and yeast. It helps the body defend itself against neurological diseases, infections, and malignancies. There are many trials looking to capitalize on the benefits of autophagy and the defense against these harmful illnesses that are affecting millions. Instead of turning to medicines and chemicals, many researchers are encouraging people to look towards a short-term restriction of food instead. This is also called intermittent fasting.

. . .

The regulation and process of autophagy involve events at a molecular level and the studies in tissue and yeast culture have added to the contemporary understanding of how it works in your body. Unfortunately, it is hard to see the process in tissues and organs that are intact, particularly the brain. It is not hard to see because of the lack of vivo mammalian models. For example, a study on a mouse provided excellent identification and evidence of the autophagy process through its production of autophago-somes and the associated protein. This study, in particular, is most often referenced marker for mammalian cells and the autophagy process. There have also been many studies on mice regarding intermittent fasting and the restrictions in vivo. Many researchers and scientists agree that autophagy is triggered during intermittent fasting and it affects many tissues and organs in the body. What is not known are its effects on the brain. Scans after two days of intermittent fasting showed no indication of autophagy in the brain. This seems to indicate that the brain is somehow more metabolically "privileged." It also indicates that a more serious stressor, such as a direct brain injury or trauma, is required to stimulate autophagy in this particular organ.

Further studies on this relationship have shown that this is not the case. One particular study on mice shows that intermittent fasting does have an effect on the autophagy process in the brain. Their approach revealed that at a certain resolution autophagosomes are increased and categorized in detail. In addition to this approach, the study published in 2010 in the scientific journal, *Autophagy*, titled "Short-term fasting induces profound neuronal autophagy," it used another method that is a bit more standard, the TEM, or transmission electron microscopy. This traditional method definitively exposed that there was a significant increase in autophagosomes in the brains of mice that were following an intermittent fasting diet. This is unlike previous conclusions, but this study clearly and definitively proves that restricting food through short-term diets, or intermittent fasting, can trigger a rapid and profound response in autophagy in the body and in the brain.

For many millions of years and across many cultures, intermittent fasting is practiced for cultural and spiritual reasons. In recent years, science has begun to explore the relationship between a person's health and intermittent fasting and have concluded there are numerous benefits to this diet plan. This "proof" may be more modern, but many cultures have long understood that there are incredible benefits when you restrict food intake for a short period of time. Prior to the study published in 2010 mentioned above, the benefits seemed to apply to your entire body, with the exception of your brain. The previous train of thought was that the brain was somehow spared the effects of short-term nutrient deprivation, including the positive benefit of autophagy. The rest of your body was able to enjoy the benefits—removed toxins, repaired cells, and refreshed immune system. While it could make sense to "spare" the brain the stress of nutrient restriction, even for a short period of time, the loss of upregulated autophagy in the brain was concerning.

Thankfully, after the study published in 2010, a contemporary understanding of intermittent fasting and autophagy has changed. Now, the scientific community understands that intermittent fasting benefits the body and the brain. There is actual evidence that there is a dramatic increase in autophagy in the brain, as well as the body when a person participates in an intermittent fasting diet plan. It is especially seen in the Purkinje and cortical neurons. This finding in 2010 led to additional studies on therapeutic applications of intermittent fasting and neurodegenerative diseases and other brain disorders. It is from this study that modern science now sees how autophagy cleanses the brain tissue and restores your brain back to the desired balance.

During the study, there were three novel conclusions and observations that are worth noting, particularly when it comes to autophagy and intermittent fasting;

1. In mammals, especially in the mice used in the study, which consumed an average diet, the researchers were able to localize and identify autophagosomes in both the Purkinje and cortical neurons.

2. In those specific neurons, when food was restricted for a short time, during the mouse's intermittent fasting period, there was a significant increase in the number of autophagosomes, which were observed alongside physical changes to the subject's characteristics as well. The results of their observations were either from the lower rate of fusion between lysosomes and autophagosomes or from the increase creation of autophagosomes. The key protein that restrains autophagy, mTOR, is reduced in the Purkinje cells of a mouse that is intermittent fasting, leading to the conclusion that the observation is from the increased production of autophagosomes. This is why the conclusion of the study explains that having more autophagosomes is from an increase in production rather than from a blockage to the maturation of the autophagosome. But it is worth noting that there is no concrete evidence of this at this time.

3. It is important to note that the changes resulting from intermittent fasting are different depending

on what cell in the brain you are looking at. This is because the process of autophagy differs from one cell type to the next in your body. This is an adaptation or evidence of evolution in the body to help meet the physiological needs of the individual cells. When autophagy is blocked in studies, it is clear that the outcome of this is determined by the tissue or cell type it was not able to respond to. For instance, in a study where the autophagy to the brain was interrupted, the brain experienced a degenerative disease. Prior to this observation, it was assumed that cells that were similar would have similar responses to an increase in autophagy, but now it is shown that this is not the case in vivo. While there was an increase in autophagosomes, the distribution and size had some differences as well as similarities in both types of cells. Because there is a difference between these similar cells, and this observation challenges the previous assumptions regarding cellular response and autophagy, it is clear more research is needed in this area. It is particularly important to study this further in relation to intermittent fasting.

There is significant clinical relevance to the discovery of intermittent fasting and its role in supporting the health of the body and the brain. It has been known for a long time that restricting the process of autophagy to the brain can lead to neurodegenerative diseases. The findings of this study described in this chapter suggest the reverse is true, too; that upregulating the production of autophagy can actually help prevent and treat neurodegenerative diseases. This process can actually help protect your brain. For example, in one study, it is shown that when a model is starved in vitro the neuronal cell lines begin to eliminate molecules that are toxic as well as mitochondria that are damaged from the affected neuron. In another study on tissue cultures, the mutant proteins responsible for Huntington disease and Parkinson's disease, a-synuclein, are able to be removed using autophagy induced by intermittent fasting.

On the other hand, there are some studies that indicate intermittent fasting improves your mind, not because of the lack of caloric intake, but because of the natural response that is triggered when your body begins to fast. In order for a drug to replicate the effects of intermittent fasting on the brain especially, it must first be able to pass through the blood-brain barrier. Once it reaches the brain intact, it then needs to stimulate the upregulation of the autophagy in the brain. And even if the drug is capable of the first two processes, scientists need to also make sure that the process and the chemicals are harmless to the subject. The medical world is years away from accomplishing something like that.

Instead, intermittent fasting is a simple, inexpensive, healthy, and reliable method for supporting the health of your body and your brain. It is an excellent alternative to taking a drug to regulate and heal your body. This is why intermittent fasting is such an attractive process for cleansing and healing your body and brain. Keep in mind, as mentioned in extended water fasting, watching your body's response is necessary. If you chronically starve your body, it can lead to autophagy inhibition instead of upregulation. This could lead to neuronal damage, rather than protection, and defeat the purpose of the practice.

One of the best things you can do, when you determine to try this method for your mental and physical health and protection, is to find a healthcare professional that can support and monitor you along the way. The effects of a short-term, intermittent fast are not as significant as the extended water fast suggested in the previous chapter, but it will still lead to stress on your body and challenges. Again, most of the challenge is mental, meaning you need to gather a good support team to encourage your progress, and you also need to prepare for your success. Begin by coming up with your purpose for intermittent fasting. Perhaps it is to support your mental clarity and protection, as the focus of this chapter describes, or maybe it is to lose weight or support your general health. Being clear about your purpose will allow you to turn back to it when you want to reach for something to eat during a fasting period. In addition, you will want to have a plan in place when those tempting times happen. There will be times when you are supposed to be fasting but you are tempted to break your fast. Determine how you will respond to these situations.

Finally, involve your support system in your goals. Maybe recruit a friend, family member, or loved one to join you on your intermittent fasting schedule. Have people support you and keep you on track. This group will be your strength when you are stressed and challenged. Once you find a schedule and break your old habits, these will not be as critical, but in the beginning, they can make the difference between successfully completing a fasting period and not. And, as mentioned before, if you do not make it through a fasting period, do not be too hard on yourself. Any step to support your health is good, so just keep going!

7

The Fasting-Mimicking Diet

Your long-term health can be improved, it is full of nutrients, and it is scientifically supported. As an alternative to the two other dieting methods mentioned in the previous chapters, this diet allows you to still eat food but enjoy the benefits of fasting. If you do not think you could take on a full fast, this is something worth trying and exploring, especially in the beginning. It is a modified type of fast. You do not cut out food completely, but you do eat a small amount that still produces the results of a fast on your body. This is something you can do a few times a week to get the best results. You can also follow this type of diet for five consecutive days to also get the most out of your efforts. The food you consume needs to have a good combination of calories, protein, and carbs, and be high in fat. Your caloric intake needs to be less than 40% of your normal limit. This is what encourages your body to enjoy the thera-peutic benefits of fasting while still supporting your body with electrolytes and nutrients and a lot less stress.

If you restrict your calories for too long or fast for too long, you can end up harming your body and counteracting your purpose. On the other hand, following a fasting-mimicking diet can be safer for longer periods of time. It can also be more effective if you follow it right.

Fasting-Mimicking Versus Fasting

One of the similarities you will find right away regarding fasting and fasting-mimicking diet is the proliferation of rumors and myths. For example, it is common to hear people claim that your muscles will deteriorate if you do this diet or fast. You may also hear claims that you will stunt your metabolism or that it is an extremely unhealthy thing to do to your body. While these facts are true for a person who is actually starving, or is cutting out, or restricting for years, it is simply not true for someone who is rationally approaching fasting or the fasting-mimicking diet. Unhealthy approaches, like actually starving yourself or severely cutting calories for months or years, can result in damage to your metabolism and are particularly dangerous for people who have other health concerns. But, especially with fasting-mimicking diets, you get all the benefits of fasting without you actually cutting out food completely. This means far less and not as severe side effects.

Benefits of Fasting-Mimicking Diet

If you return to the previous chapters outlining the benefits of autophagy and the benefits of fasting in relation to autophagy, you could basically "copy and paste" them here. They are essentially the same:

- Refresh and renew your immune system
- Increased removal and recycling of damaged or dysfunctional cells or cellular parts, including cancerous and infectious particles
- An upregulated autophagy process throughout your body
- Ketosis lowers the amount of fat tissue in the body
- Less oxidative stress and C-reactive proteins in the body, most likely because of the autophagy process
- Longevity promoted through increased expression of your genes
- Improved brain development, protection, prevention, and performance through upregulated autophagy as well as more BDNF, or brain-derived neurotrophic factors. BDNF helps the brain grow new neurons and current neurons survive longer.
- Lowered glucose levels, better regenerative markers, and homeostatic stem cell levels

- Lowered risk for various diseases such as cancer, diabetes, and neurodegenerative diseases like Parkinson's and Alzheimer's.

By mirroring or "ticking" your body into thinking it is fasting, your body can trigger and stimulate these responses in your body so you can enjoy these benefits. What you are also doing is making sure that your body continually receives the nutrients it needs and craves every day.

How the Process Works

As you begin your research into fasting-mimicking diet plans, it is important to start in the same manner as the other two methods listed earlier; start with your "why" or your purpose. Be clear about why you are doing this diet and what you want to get from it. If it is to lower your risk of cancer, how will you make sure you are supporting this health goal and know what you are doing is working? If you want to improve your mental focus, how will you measure this for success? Start with a purpose, develop a plan, and determine how you will know it is "working" for you. This preparation will make sure you are ready for the challenges that inevitably lie ahead.

. . .

Most research on the fasting-mimicking diet suggests that five or more days are best to get your glucose levels low enough that your body enters ketosis, or begins burning fat for fuel instead of glucose. This means you want your glucose index below 1.0. For some people, especially those that have done this diet a few times, they will only need to follow it for three or four days to see the results, while others may always need to follow it for six or seven days. Do not extend this diet past seven days at a time to best support your general health. You can do this diet a couple times in a year or even once a month. The more you do it, the better your body will be at switching over into ketosis and the faster and more results you will see.

It is a good idea to measure your biomarkers to track your outcomes. You can do this with conducting labs before and after the fast or by measuring your blood glucose and ketones throughout your fasting period. Track these markers daily along with your weight to determine if the fast and caloric plan is working well for you. You may want to adjust your caloric intake up or down depending on these biomarkers. You can have a healthcare professional help you draw labs before and after your fast, or you can get at-home blood glucose and ketone test kit to monitor for yourself. An at-home bathroom scale is also helpful in this process.

. . .

As you begin to prepare for your fast, prepare your environment appropriately. This means alerting your support system of what you are doing, as well as others around you that you will come in contact with during the fast. Tell them your purpose for it and why their support is helpful to you. Having someone who is doing it with you and is keeping the same schedule can be helpful as well. Also, clear out snacks and "junk food" from your house, car, and work. Remove any and all temptations, especially during your fast. Plan to get enough rest over the several days of your fast. You will probably notice a drop in energy levels as your body tries to adjust to the reduction in glucose energy supply. If you prepare for this with enough time blocked out for a good night sleep, and maybe a nap or two here and there, you will be much happier during the process. This does not mean you need to avoid daily activity or physical activity altogether. Light to moderate physical activity is good for you during this time and can actually speed up the process. Avoid strenuous actions, like long distance running or weight training, but a nice walk or yoga can be beneficial.

Some Facts To Know

As you begin this diet plan, you may want to consider "easing" into it by eating foods with higher caloric content, about 50% of your total intake, and then bringing it down towards the remaining few days to between 35% and 40% of your normal caloric intake. Also, stock up on snacks and foods that are easy to grab, digest, and are satisfying in small amounts. You can look into the brand ProLon, which has developed prepackaged foods for the fasting-mimicking diet. You can get the entire kit of food designed for a five-day fasting-mimicking diet plan. They are plant-based and adjusted for a normal, healthy adult woman and man's caloric intake. One day includes meals like a tea and mixed nut bar for breakfast, kale crackers, and soup for lunch, olives for a snack, and soup for dinner. The process is meant to take the prep and stress out of the diet so you can just enjoy the benefits.

Of course, you do not need to buy something pre-packaged to enjoy the benefits of the fasting-mimicking diet. A ketogenic diet, which is low in carbs, is great to follow on a fasting-mimicking diet, and just requires you to space out your calories appropriately during the fasting period. It is a wise idea to plan meals for your entire fast so there is nothing to think about during the five or so days.

A typical macro breakdown for a fasting-mimicking diet on the first day includes:

- Carbs: 34%
- Protein: 10%
- Fat: 56%

After the first day, adjust for the following macros:

- Carbs: 47%
- Protein: 9%
- Fat: 44%

These macros are different than the ketogenic diet, so adjust accordingly if you decide to follow that meal plan while restricting your calories during your fasting period.

You are not restricted from having some conveniences during your fasting-mimicking diet, either. For example, you can have a cup of black coffee, with no sugar added, or tea. You can add coconut oil if you want, but you need to track the macros appropriately. You do not need to drink these beverages if you do not want to, and just stick to water, but they are available should you choose.

Also, you may want to consider taking a supplement on your fasting days to make sure your body is getting all the required nutrients. This is especially beneficial as you learn how to balance your plate with a lower caloric limit. If you are already following a balanced and healthy diet, you may not need to supplement, but for those who need it, consider the following:

- Salt and magnesium to replenish electrolyte loss
- Liver tablets (grass-fed) to support micronutrients
- BCAA's or branch chain amino acids to prevent tissue loss, especially if you are working out heavily during your fasting days
- Powdered greens to offer a dose of micronutrients
- Algal oil or cod liver oil for omega-3

Ketosis and Fasting-mimicking Diets

Before you start the ketogenic diet, it may be a good idea to start with a fasting-mimicking diet. It can help get your body into ketosis faster when you begin the ketogenic diet. In addition, focusing on ketogenic foods can help you remain in ketosis for the length of your diet. This means you will want to adjust your macros to something more like this:

- Carbs: 5-10%
- Protein: 20-25%
- Fat: 70-80%

On the ketogenic diet, the best bet is to choose something high in fat every time. This includes:

- Avocados
- Grass-fed butter
- Bone Broth
- Coconut milk
- Coconut oil

8

Bonus! Weight Loss and Autophagy

So you want to lose weight? Maybe it is your primary reason for looking into autophagy, or it is an additional benefit you are excited about. Hopefully, by now, you recognize that through autophagy, one of the great benefits is that you can finally get rid of that stubborn ten (or more) pounds that seem to never leave. And you can do this alongside a healthy process that is natural and beneficial to your body. How many diet plans that promise you to lose weight can say they also help your brain function better, prevent diseases, and make your skin look younger? How many can say there is a chance you can live longer because of this plan? Not many. But when you trigger autophagy in your body, you can get all of that along with losing weight.

Now, the caveat here is that you have to have weight to lose. This only works for people who are not at their ideal weight for the age and height. This is because your autophagy process will drop you down to this ideal weight range, but no lower unless you force it, and then you lose the benefits of autophagy. Instead, you should focus on getting to that healthy weight and let your body continue to regulate your health from there. You can follow any of the methods mentioned earlier in this book to help you lose weight, but one of them that is particularly beneficial for women is intermittent fasting. But this does not mean it does not work well for men as well!

For example, in a study conducted at the University of Florida by Dr. Stephen Anton, the participants who fasted for 24 hours every other day saw notable weight loss compared to their counterparts. And these results were replicated ten times; each time those that participated in the intermittent fasting protocol saw significant weight loss. And alongside the weight loss, the study indicated several other health benefits these participants enjoyed from "switching up" their metabolism.

This switch is when your body moves from burning glucose to fat. You no longer rely on glucose and blood sugar to fuel your body and instead look to fatty acids and ketones. This is how you can get at those stubborn fat pockets that never seem to go away, no matter what diet you have tried before. When you are wanting to gain muscle and burn fat, you want to turn to your fat stores to burn off. It is the best and most natural fuel for your body. Once you begin burning your body fat, you no longer start storing it. As you run through your stores of fat, the food that does come in is burned before it can linger. This is why and how you lose weight and keep it off through autophagy. Your body is programmed to do this at its most basic, cellular level, and will thank you when you do it by being at its healthy weight, clearest skin, focused brain, and overall healthy body. You will not get as sick as often because your immune system is functioning at optimal levels. Your body is constantly targeting, repairing, removing, and regenerating cells, tissues, and organs while you fast and sleep. You are giving it the time and space to be able to do this.

Of course, this is more of a lifestyle than a temporary or "fad" diet. Triggering autophagy and entering into ketosis needs to be consistent so your body is constantly supporting your health and weight goals. In addition, once you lose the weight and drop to your healthy weight range, as you continue to burn fat and heal your body, you will be able to lose a few more pounds as you replace more fat stores with muscles and healthy tissue. You can only enjoy this benefit if you keep up the plan. This is where some plans can be too restrictive and can lead to backsliding. You can experience short-term weight loss but then fail to continue the diet and you gain back all the weight, and often more than you lost. In one statistic, it is estimated that more than 95% of women who lose weight through an extreme diet was unable to keep the weight off. The study also indicated that the health and weight of these women were worse after the diet than it was before. You do not want to be in that "boat," so make sure you choose a method for triggering the autophagy that is sustainable for you. Or choose a plan that you think you can work your way into and stay there for a length of time.

It is great to experience rapid weight loss and improved health, but you also want it to be realistic for the long-term. This may mean you start off "slow," triggering autophagy once or twice a week through a day of intermittent fasting and a day of intense exercise, or you choose a stretch of five days one month to try the fasting-mimicking diet. The goal is to start by experimenting with the different options until you decide a process that works for you and then stick with it. That is how you can enjoy the long-term results possible with an upregulated autophagy process.

Thankfully, in most instances, you can still enjoy your favorite treats and foods on your "off" days. In all three methods described in this book, none of them said you never could have a piece of cake, glass of wine, beer, or a piece of pizza again. In fact, you can enjoy those when you want, as long as it is not on a day you are fasting. Of course, your results are better if you minimize these "treats," but take a moment to think about how much easier it will be on yourself when you say, "I cannot have that donut today, but I will save it for tomorrow when I am no longer fasting." Or, "I am not going to go out to lunch today, but will take a walk outside instead. When I am done with my current triggering process I am going to make sure to treat myself to a nice dinner out."

If you want to combine the ketogenic diet with intermittent fasting, you can restrict food for 12 to 24 hours completely and then cycle in higher-levels of protein. Doing this sends your body from deprivation to intense intake, activating your autophagy process more frequently. The fasting process lowers your glucose and then the protein comes in it triggers it starting autophagy.

There is no hard and fast rule for how often you should be triggering your autophagy response for weight loss and health. This will most likely depend on you and your preferences. Some research suggests for the best results you should conduct and intermittent fast on three non-consecutive days during the week. You can rotate the days or keep them the same from week to week. This may not be feasible with your schedule or it can fit in well. If three days is too much, consider alternating it so you have a couple days one week and three days another. If you are following the fasting-mimicking diet to lose weight and trigger autophagy, aim for about five days on the diet plan about once a month. If this is too much, plan to follow the diet at least once a quarter or twice a year. Extended water fasting can be done for one to 20 days, depending on your body and needs. If you choose to follow this method, you should do so under the guidance of a professional and adjust or introduce food in when necessary.

If you want to follow the method below, it can help you lose weight and keep it off quickly. You will first begin by choosing three days out of the week that you will call your "low" days. These are designed to trigger your autophagy by stressing your cells through nutrient restriction. The remaining four days of the week are your "high" days and will begin to inhibit your autophagy response. The "low" days will include an overnight fast totaling 16 hours. For the last eight hours of the day, cut back on your protein intake significantly. Try to eat less than 25 grams of protein in this time frame. On your "high" days, enjoy. No restrictions!

The purpose of this meal plan is to increase weight loss, trigger autophagy, and support a long-term eating plan for the best results. You are activating and inhibiting autophagy constantly through this process. You need to have the "low" days with some intake after a fast because your body requires nutrients to survive. It cannot stay in a constant state of deprivation. This is what leads to starvation, the inhibition of autophagy, and eventually death. Also, restricting protein completely is not good for you either. Cutting it out altogether can lead to immune diseases and increased health risks, as well as muscle deterioration. This cyclical nature of the plan allows your body to get what it needs while also benefiting from the activated autophagy.

In addition to the minimal "low" days during the week, you get to choose when they will be! Of course, the "low" days need to remain non-consecutive, but you can select what is best for you based on your schedule. And they do not need to be the same from week to week. Also, on your "high" days, do not hold yourself back from what you want. You may notice over time that you tend to select healthier foods and are eating less, but that should come naturally and not be forced. It is this approach that helps keep this diet plan sustainable. A word of advice on choosing your "low" days is to avoid choosing a weekend for a "low." This is because most events and special treats occur on Saturday and Sunday. Consider Monday, Wednesday, and Friday as "low" days. This means every weekend you can indulge, as well as on Tuesdays and Thursdays!

To help further illustrate, here is a breakdown of what this could look like for you and your weight loss journey:

Day

Restriction

Sunday

High- No limits!

Monday

Low- fast overnight for a total of 16 hours, minimal protein intake not to exceed 25 grams for eight hours

Tuesday

High- No limits!

Wednesday

Low- fast overnight for a total of 16 hours, minimal protein intake not to exceed 25 grams for eight hours

Thursday

High- No limits!

Friday

Low- fast overnight for a total of 16 hours, minimal protein intake not to exceed 25 grams for eight hours

Saturday

High- No limits!

Make sure to customize this plan to fit your life. That is how you can best use autophagy triggering to fit into your life for a long time. Move your days and times around until you get a mix that makes sense for you. Or try another method mentioned in the book. There are plenty of options available to you for losing weight with autophagy. You just need to start triggering it!

Conclusion

Thank for making it through to the end of *Autophagy: Body's Natural Intelligence for Anti-Aging and Healing – Intermittent Fasting for Weight Loss & Self-Cleansing.* Let's hope it was informative and able to provide you with all of the tools you need to achieve your goals whatever they may be.

The next step on your journey, now that you have learned about what autophagy, is learn how it impacts your body in a variety of ways and determine what you are going to do with this information. Are you going to use it to help lose weight, protect your brain, reset your immune system, clear your skin, and support your general health? If so, how are you planning on doing it? There are different options presented to you in this book. You can choose what you think will work best for you and get started.

Below is a step-by-step guide for getting started:

1. Determine why you want to trigger autophagy. Is it for weight loss? Or is it to help prevent disease and illness? Be clear about your "why" and your purpose.

2. Enlist people to support you on your journey. Tell your loved ones, friends, and family about what you want to do and why. Ask them to support and encourage you as you experiment with finding a process that works for you. Maybe even find another person to embark on this journey with you!

3. Choose or develop a strategy that you think will work best in your life. Look into adding intense exercise into your week, partake in extended water fasting, intermittent fasting, fasting-mimicking or even the intermittent fasting and protein cycling plan presented in the last chapter. There are numerous combinations and options you can choose from, including type and frequency. Take a moment to look at your calendar and determine what you think will realistically fit in.

4. Clear out temptations and distractions from your kitchen, car, and work. Anything that does not fit with your strategy needs to go. Plan out some healthy meals that fit with your plan, gather up snacks that you can grab on the run, and prepare for your first trial.

5. Get started! Set a day to begin, tell your support
   system, and start.

Remember, you do not need to always accomplish your goals. If you do not make it through your first try, do not give up! This is just the beginning. Learn from the first attempt and adjust to better suit your situation the next time. Each time you give your plan a try, learn from what works and what does not, and adjust for next time. You are making great strides for your health, and each attempt is furthering you on this journey. Keep it up!

Finally, if you found this book useful in any way, a review on Amazon is always appreciated!